THE PRINCIPAL

DISEASES OF INDIA,

BRIEFLY DESCRIBED

THE PRINCIPAL

DISEASES OF INDIA,

BRIEFLY DESCRIBED:

WITH

HINTS ON THE DUTIES OF MEDICAL OFFICERS IN THAT COUNTRY.

BY

CHARLES ALEX. GORDON, M. D.

STAFF SURGEON, SECOND CLASS.

GYAN

Published by

GYAN

Gyan Publishing House
5, Ansari Road
Daryaganj, New Delhi-110002
Phone: 011-47034999, 9811692060
E-mail: books@gyanbooks.com

Distribution Network
gyanbooks.com
India, USA, Canada, UK, Australia

ISBN: 978-81-212-7531-6 (PB)
First Published, 1847

2nd Impression 2024

Printed at: Gyan Press, Delhi.

THE PRINCIPAL DISEASES OF INDIA, BRIEFLY DESCRIBED
Author: CHARLES ALEX. GORDON

THE PRINCIPAL

DISEASES OF INDIA,

BRIEFLY DESCRIBED:

WITH

HINTS ON THE DUTIES OF MEDICAL OFFICERS IN THAT COUNTRY.

BY

CHARLES ALEX. GORDON, M.D.

STAFF SURGEON, SECOND CLASS.

LONDON:

TRELAWNEY WM. SAUNDERS,

6, CHARING CROSS.

1847.

PREFACE.

THE following brief sketch of the principal diseases to which Europeans in India are liable, has been written with the intention of stating as concisely as possible the result of my own experience during the time I had the honour to serve with one of H. M.'s Regiments in that country.

I have endeavoured to exclude all theoretical matter, and to give a plain statement of the ordinary phenomena of those diseases, together with the remedies which I found to be most successful in their treatment.

In this way a ready means of reference has been obtained, which it is hoped may prove useful to the junior members of the profession; especially as in larger and more elaborate medical works, the necessary discussion of various opinions tends frequently to confuse rather than to enlighten those who have had no opportunity of judging for themselves at the bed-side of the sick.

The observations for the guidance of Medical Officers, have been introduced, because I am aware, from experience, of the difficulty Surgeons frequently have to encounter in becoming acquainted with the system of official communication with the departments in India, it being radically different from the method adopted both in the United Kingdom and in the Colonies; so that even old and experienced Surgeons often find themselves very much at the mercy of the Subordinate Department for some time after their arrival in the country.

Being on the eve of proceeding abroad, circumstances have induced me to hurry the publication of this volume, and have rendered its revision impracticable. I trust, therefore, some allowance will be made on that account for whatever imperfections and omissions may be discovered in it.

C. A. G.

LONDON, Dec. 1846.

CONTENTS.

HINTS ON THE DUTIES

OF MEDICAL OFFICERS IN INDIA.

Suggestions on landing, either alone or with troops—Head money—Pay—Surplus medicine—Retrenchments—Junior Officers often left in charge of Regiment—Consequent duties—Stores—Subordinate Medical Establishment—Their duties—Supply of Medicines, &c.—Committees—Returns—Change of Quarters—Materials for conveyance of sick by water and by land—Concurrence of Commanding Officer—Consequences of Hospital being placed in rear on march—Suggestions for obviating the inconvenience—Routine duty—Relative position of Commanding Officer and Surgeon.

NOTWITHSTANDING the numerous works that have been written on subjects relating to India, the Medical Officer of H. M. Service, for the first time arriving in that country, often finds on landing that he is quite at a loss what to do. It is therefore anticipated that the few general hints now offered will prove to be acceptable to the junior members of the profession, whose lot it is to serve in the East.

When an officer, of whatever denomination, arrives in India, the first thing to be done by him is to proceed direct to the office of the Brigade Major, and there insert his name and date of landing in a book which is kept for that purpose. The Medical Officer is next to proceed to the office of the Inspector General of H. M.'s Hospitals, to whom it is etiquette to report himself personally; but should that not be in his power, it is his duty to write officially. In case of his having had the good fortune to obtain charge of troops on the voyage from England, it will be necessary, at the same time that he reports his arrival, to transmit a statement of the strength and constitution of the detachment, as well as a report of the state of the sick, and of the casualties that may have occurred at sea. He is then to forward at an early opportunity the Journal and Instruments which he received from the India House in London, to the Secretary at the Medical Board in Calcutta; from whom he will receive a certificate (if the Journal be properly kept) which will entitle him to the "Head money," amounting to 15s. sterling for each man and officer, and 10s. 6d. for each woman and child, landed; which sum the Company very liberally pay at the rate of 1s. 10d. per rupee. The Medical Officer must make up his mind, however, to submit to some of "the delays of office" before he can receive his money, although it is certain enough to be paid after a time.

Until an officer joins his regiment and balances his accounts with the Paymaster, he obtains his pay from the Company merely on account; and at some stations there is so much difficulty attending this arrangement, that it is necessary for an officer who wishes to draw money to write officially to the Major General commanding; to whom he must explain the circumstances under which he is desirous to obtain a certain sum from the Paymaster of that district.

It is absolutely necessary that every officer should have obtained a certificate of last pay from the Regimental Agents in England, which certificate is to be appended to the first bill that is forwarded to the Paymaster of the Queen's troops in India.

It is very rarely that the amount of the bill can be obtained until several days after it has been rendered, as it must first be passed by the Audit Office. After a time, however, the authorized amount will be paid; or in the event of the drawer having proceeded to a distant station in the meantime, an order on the Collector will be forwarded to it, or to any intermediate station, if he request the Paymaster to do so.

When an officer is ordered to proceed by water, or to march from one station to another at a considerable distance, he ought invariably to write to the Paymaster of the Queen's troops, to forward a certificate of last pay to await his arrival at some intermediate post town; as by that means a great deal of unpleasant reference to General Officers of stations may be avoided. Officers serving in Bengal with troops, however, are usually sent to Chinsurah, a station situated on the right bank of the river Hooghly, about thirty miles up from Calcutta, where there is a depôt of Queen's troops, commanded by an officer who has had considerable experience in the country; junior officers will therefore generally find his advice very useful, when they are not too proud to confess their own ignorance, by asking his counsel on matters of which they cannot be expected to know anything.

When the Medical Officer arriving with troops has some surplus medicine left, he will frequently be able to dispose of it to the master of the vessel; or else a druggist will always be ready to purchase it, although, in that case, at a price far under its real value. It is recommended to every person, however, whether he belong to the medical profession or not, to have a small stock of medicine in his own possession; as the severe diseases to which Europeans are subject in India, attack without much previous warning, and in many instances they attain to a fatal height, before a medical man can attend and get his prescription prepared at the regimental hospital.

The preceding remarks on the subject of Officers' pay in India, have extended to some length, as it has been frequently observed that those who have never been in that country entertain the idea that rupees are served out to the servants of the Company in a sort of wholesale manner; whereas there really is, at times, a very great difficulty in obtaining the amount to which one is actually entitled. The "Pay and allowances" are divided into such a number of items, such as "Queen's pay," "Batta," "Tentage," "Gratuity," &c., that while an officer is on detachment duty he is constantly liable to have some portion of his bill *retrenched* by the Audit Office; and although he generally recovers the amount after a great deal of correspondence, still many officers who have been *retrenched* for small sums allow them to pass unnoticed rather than be at all the trouble of a more or less protracted correspondence.

Although the medical establishment in India is considered very complete, there is nevertheless a difficulty at times in obtaining the assistance of an officer of any considerable standing. Accordingly one of two or three years' service is occasionally called upon to take charge of a large detachment, or even of a regiment; it is therefore no matter of surprise that a person of so little experience should feel at a loss, when first placed in a situation of such responsibility.

In such a case, he generally finds that all the necessary stores have been laid in by his predecessor; and that he is only required to examine the correctness of the lists of articles which have been furnished to him, and to exchange receipts for the same; forwarding one copy to the Superintending Surgeon of the district, and reporting the circumstance of his having assumed charge, to the Inspector of Her Majesty's Hospitals. When, however, a detachment marches from a depôt, or when a regiment first lands in the country, it becomes necessary for the officer in charge to procure the requisite stores. This is done by indents or requisitions, which have to be forwarded to the offices of the Superintending Surgeon and Commissariat Officer; but as the most explicit instructions upon this point are contained in the "Bengal Medical Code," with which every hospital is supplied by the Superintending Surgeon of the district, it is only desirable to mention that the indents should be made out in strict conformity to the rules therein laid down.

Every hospital in India is furnished by the Company with a subordinate medical establishment, such as a steward, apothecary, apprentices, and hospital servants, for the payment of all of whom the Surgeon is responsible; but as they are paid by the Commissariat Baboo of the station, all that is required of the Surgeon is to see that each of them signs the acquittance roll, and then to append his own name, after having ascertained that the whole is correct.

It may be remarked, in justice to the members of the Bengal Subordinate Medical Department, that they are really a most useful and intelligent class of men. They are all Europeans by one or both parents; and although but few have ever been out of the country, they are nevertheless tolerably well educated, and usually understand the ordinary routine duties of a Hospital.

The Apothecaries have charge of the medicines, assist the Surgeon in making out his returns to the Queen's Inspector of Hospitals, dispense the prescriptions, and see that the medicines are administered as ordered. They also attend to the calls of patients in Hospital, and to those who come for admission, until one of the medical officers can be sent for. The Steward on the other hand, has charge of the clothing, keeps the account of the Hospital expenditure, is responsible for the stores of every description, with the exception of the medicines, and furnishes the returns of his department to the Superintending Surgeon, who is always a Company's officer.

Medicines and Instruments are obtained by half-yearly indents as in England, and Hospital clothing is served out once a year, that is, in October; but before the Superintending Surgeon will pass the indents for these stores, he requires that a Committee shall report that the old are unserviceable, and have been rendered so by fair wear and tear, and not by carelessness on the part of those who have had charge of them. It is therefore advisable when any articles have been lost, or an accident occurs, to report the circumstance to the Commanding Officer, who will order a Committee to assemble and inquire into it. Committees are so common in India, that it would appear as if an officer were capable of giving an opinion on every possible article, whether medicines, clothes, tents, boats, camels, elephants, roads, in fact every thing. The object of referring matters to the decision of a Committee, is to remove the responsibility from a particular individual, although many amusing anecdotes are related in India of the decisions of such committees: for instance I have been told by an officer, that he was once a member of one appointed to examine some commissariat camels, the whole of which were rejected because they had marks of "broken knees."

In the event of any medicine being required between the regular periods at which requisitions for a supply are forwarded, it is customary to transmit an "Emergent Indent" to the Superintending Surgeon, who will immediately forward the quantity required by dâk or post, for every one must admit that the Indian Government is most liberal in providing for its sick soldiers.

Such articles as are produced in the country can usually be obtained from the Commissariat Department without any further reference, provided that no more than the regulated allowance be required; but when there has been occasion to exceed this, it becomes necessary to have the indent sanctioned by the Superintending Surgeon.

Among the returns to be rendered by a medical officer in charge of European troops, are: 1. A daily state to the Commanding officer. 2. A weekly state to the Superintending Surgeon of the district. 3. A monthly return of sick to the Inspector General of H.M.'s troops. 4. A monthly return according to another form, to the Superintending Surgeon. 5. A monthly return of hospital stoppages to the Paymaster, if with a regiment; and to the Commanding Officer, if with a detachment. 6. A quarterly return of sick and wounded to the Inspector General; to which is to be appended a detailed medical report of the occurrences in the regiment or detachment, during the period embraced by it. 7. A similar return to the Superintending Surgeon, to which is to be annexed a report of the number of sick, the number of hospital diets consumed during the period, as well as a tabular return showing the expenditure of wine, beer, and spirits, the quantity remaining in store, and the quantity required for the ensuing quarter. 8. Half-yearly returns of medicines; and on the 1st of October, a return of clothing, as already stated. 9. An annual return of sick and wounded, with detailed medical report of the occurrences in the regiment, is to be sent within fourteen days after 1st of April, to the Inspector General of Queen's Troops; and by a late order, a copy of it must likewise be transmitted to the Superintending Surgeon. 10. A sanatory report has to be furnished annually, according to a form supplied by the War Office to the Officer commanding the regiment. 11. A half-yearly return, showing the state of vaccination in the regiment. 12. A line of the No. 3 return is to be filled in annually, reckoning from the date of the arrival of the regiment in the country; in which the following points are to be enumerated among others, viz., the stations occupied by the regiment during the year; the average strength of the corps; the number of recruits and volunteers who have joined; the number who have become non-effective; and the average sick and ratio of mortality, stating also the mortality from each disease which has proved fatal. This return is very complete in itself, showing at one view all the changes which have taken place in a regiment during its term of foreign service. While abroad, it is to be forwarded to the Inspector General, and on the return of the regiment to England it is to be filled up, the totals being given in the last column, and forwarded to the Director General. In addition to these there are other reports which are required of a Medical Officer; for instance, when troops are on the march or proceeding by water, it is necessary to transmit to the Inspector General a diary, in which every particular respecting the troops must be given; and when an epidemic such as cholera breaks out, it will be necessary to forward a daily state of the patients who are suffering from it; also whenever we pass a large station, it is etiquette, if not our duty, to wait upon the Senior Medical Officer with a state of the sick for the information of the General Officer commanding.

All these returns will no doubt appear very complicated, although they are by no means so in reality; for by ordinary attention a person will readily fall into the routine duty connected with a hospital.

The conveyance of the sick, when a regiment or detachment changes quarters, is another subject of interest to the Medical Officer.

The usual period at which regiments and detachments change quarters in India is August, if they are conveyed by water; and October or November, which is the commencement of the cold season, when they proceed by land; and as the climate, particularly in the upper provinces, is very agreeable until the latter half of March, troops frequently march a distance of six or eight hundred miles in the cold season; only halting on Sundays, and on their arrival at a large station, for the purpose of laying in commissariat supplies and to rest the cattle.

Without commenting on the arrangements of the Honourable East India Company, it cannot but be observed that European troops are always more healthy on the march than during the passage by water; and the experience of the last few years shows what a melancholy loss has been sustained in men and officers by regiments which have landed in the country during the rainy season.

When troops are ordered to proceed by water,

tonnage is procured for the sick by indenting upon the Commissariat through the Superintending Surgeon; but as the regulations upon this point contained in the "Pay and Audit Regulations," and "Medical Code," were not so explicit formerly as could have been desired, it will be well to forward an indent through the Regimental Commanding Officer and Quarter Master; as by so doing any disagreeable collision with the Commanding Officer is avoided, which might otherwise arise from following the "Code" without referring to the "Pay and Audit Regulations," the latter being the book of reference upon financial points with all departments except the Medical.

When troops proceed by land, hospital tents are provided agreeably to indents countersigned by the Commanding Officer, and sent to the Quarter Master; carriage being provided by the Commissariat Department. Doolies are also supplied by the Commissariat in the proportion of ten per cent. when a regiment is ordered upon service; and of course in a smaller proportion when merely changing quarters. In the latter case additional doolies can always be provided at some of the larger stations through which the route is certain to lie; or when diseases render it unsafe for patients to accompany the corps, they can be left in an European hospital. The necessary proportion of doolie bearers, tent pitchers, &c., are in like manner procured and paid by the Commissariat Department; so that after sending in correct indents, a medical man has really very little to do with the arrangements arising from the departure of a corps from a station. So liberal are the Company with respect to hospital affairs, that the authorised allowances for accommodation and attendance of the sick are generally more than sufficient, except in cases where an epidemic suddenly makes its appearance among the men, and even then every facility is afforded for making the necessary arrangements for such an increase of sick. It generally happens that the sick list decreases when a corps has been for a short time on the move, and particularly should it be marching; in which case it will be advisable to part with the surplus doolies, or an extra boat, if we are proceeding by water; as so long as the corps remains in the Company's territory, any supplies that may be required can always be obtained; and when proceeding on service the authorised supply is of course laid in at once, and not parted with under any circumstances until the corps returns to quarters.

In lower Bengal, the only means of transport available when troops proceed by land, consists of hackeries or native carts, drawn by two or four bullocks, according to their size; but being very ricketty they constantly break down, or the miserable animals attached to them give up from sheer fatigue and bad feeding; so that this kind of carriage is extremely objectionable, and only to be recommended when no better can be procured. Camels ought always to be procured if possible; and when two or three elephants can be obtained for the carriage of the hospital, they ought to be by all means; for they are always certain to be upon the encamping ground in time, whatever may be the nature of the country over which they travel.

When on the march the regulations of the Service order the Hospital establishment to follow in rear of the column, and generally speaking that is without doubt the proper place for the sick; but while in the Company's dominions in the East Indies, there is nothing to fear from the natives, for a single European may travel there with more security than he might anticipate in some parts of the United Kingdom. On the score of safety then, it is not absolutely necessary to have the sick protected by a guard; and there are so many advantages to be gained by sending them in front, that most regiments which have been some time in the country, invariably do so.

When the sick are kept in rear of the column, the road is apt to get so blocked up with the baggage and camp-followers, and accidents are of such frequent occurrence among the cattle and hackeries, that the hospital tents are seldom pitched and the sick made comfortable under this arrangement, before the heat of the day has increased to such a degree as to be very prejudicial, were they furnished with no other protection than the open doolies. This evil may be obviated by sending forward one or two of the hospital tents on the previous evening, the cooks, &c. over night, and the sick an hour or so before the main column. The road will then be unobstructed, and the sick will be in readiness for the surgeon to pay his visit, and for their breakfast, while the morning is yet pleasantly cool. Very urgent cases can of course be attended to before they start, and for further convenience it will be advisable to have a moderate quantity of medicine, instruments, bandages, &c. in a couple of petaras, carried by a banghy-badar, so as to be constantly at hand in the event of an accident occurring; and the empty doolies should be kept close in rear, for the accommodation of those who may fall out, in consequence of sudden illness or over fatigue.

It must be recollected that these observations are

only applicable while in the Company's territory; for after it is left, and actual service has commenced, the sick as well as the healthy must "rough it." Still the medical man may, by a little management, render those under his immediate charge tolerably comfortable; and to one not acquainted with a soldier's life in India, the facilities which all have for making themselves happy while marching, may appear surprising; notwithstanding "the getting up in the middle of the night, and having no houses to sleep in."

On the river, it is but right that the hospital boats should bring up the rear of the fleet; for while proceeding up the country, a boat in which a person is taken suddenly ill can readily drop astern; and the fleet being always compact when coming down, notice can be passed from one boat to another, for the Surgeon's *orderly dingy* to convey the person to hospital immediately. It is of comparatively little consequence, however, so far as the personal comfort of the sick is concerned, in what part of the fleet they may be. Nor does it signify whether the boats are moving or not; the hospital establishment being always recognized by having a black flag at the stern of each boat. The boat of the medical officer is similarly distinguishable by a particular flag at the mast head; so that there is never any difficulty in keeping up the communication; unless the fleet happens to be scattered by some of the violent storms which so frequently occur upon the Ganges, rendering a voyage from Calcutta to Cawnpore or Allahabad far more dangerous than one round the Cape to England.

The breakfasts of the men are always served out in the morning, and the Medical Officer has sufficient time to visit the sick before the fleet starts. As the Commanding Officer's boat is the first to move, on the advance being sounded, so it is the first to come to, on the halt being called; and he generally brings up sufficiently early in the afternoon, to enable all the boats to be at their *lagowing ground* before night closes in. It must be obvious, however, that there are many inconveniences attending a voyage up or down the Ganges, and that it is not always possible to visit the men so regularly as when on the march. Many allowances must therefore doubtless be made; but generally speaking the duties of the Surgeon can be carried on regularly, and with less actual discomfort than might at first sight be apprehended.

When detachments are sent up the country by water, they are generally placed under the command of an officer of considerable experience; consequently a medical officer has seldom to interfere with any of his arrangements. Very frequently the halting ground will be of directly opposite character to what a surgeon would desire; but when the banks of the river are at times high and precipitous to the extent of many miles, and in others low and swampy, the Medical Officer must be content to halt at places the very appearances of which indicate fever and cholera. It is no doubt in consequence of these high alluvial banks in some places, and the immense extent of surrounding swamp at others, that few, if any, detachments have ever been known to escape a more or less severe visitation of these diseases, after proceeding for a considerable distance by water. All the recommendations that can be given in connexion with this point, are to choose a dry open ground, when it is available; to avoid as much as possible remaining a night to leeward of a high bank; and when we are unavoidably obliged to lagow in a bad position, to be off again at the earliest opportunity.

It is frequently asserted that the Surgeon of a regiment is totally independent of his Commanding Officer. From the very nature of his professional duties the Surgeon has, no doubt, much less intercourse with him than any of the other officers, they being daily and hourly in communication, either on parade or in the orderly room, upon various subjects relating to the men under their immediate command; whereas the Surgeon forwards the greater number of his returns, and carries on the business of the hospital, without reference to the Commanding Officer. Still, however, as the Commanding Officer must exert his authority over every department of the regiment, and is bound by the regulations of the service to visit the hospital at stated periods, and to inquire into the different points regarding the comfort of the sick, the medical department becomes virtually as much under his superintendance as any other, although it is generally left to the entire control of the Surgeon. It is a remarkable circumstance, and one which is exceedingly to be regretted, that there should be so little cordiality between the Commanding Officers and Surgeons of regiments serving in India; and while it would no doubt be difficult to say who is most to blame, it is easy to conclude that neither are immaculate.

Duty can never be conducted in a satisfactory manner where this unpleasant state of affairs exists; it therefore should be the object of all, to give that mutual accommodation in their official communication with each other which, at the same time that it does not interfere with the strictest performance of duty, renders it agreeable to all whom it associates together.

THE PRINCIPAL
DISEASES OF INDIA.

CHAPTER I.

INTRODUCTION.

Introduction—Effect of climate—Temperate and intemperate habits—Luxurious living—Effect of diet on Natives—Seasoning Fever.

THE most important diseases to which Europeans residing in the East Indies are liable, are, Remittent Fever, Dysentery, Cholera, Hepatitis, and Apoplexy; and the experience of all medical men tends to prove that these diseases make their greatest ravages among persons who have lately arrived in the country, the liability to be attacked by them being reduced after the individual has resided for some time there.

The greatest mortality always occurs among those who have been less than five or six years in the country; and of these, persons who have been in India less than three years, are most liable to the endemic diseases. The ranks of our regiments on first arriving in the country, appear to be weeded of all the delicate men they contain; any predisposition to visceral disease that had existed, being roused into a state of activity by the change of climate. On the other hand, it would also appear as if nature had endowed some persons with constitutions, to the health of which an Indian climate is conducive; it being well known that many people, who are constantly invalids at home, become stout and robust after residing in India for a short time.

It is generally supposed in England that it is only the drunken and the dissipated among whom the great mortality in India occurs; while it is as universally imagined that "water drinkers" are almost completely exempt from disease. Such were the ideas entertained by me before going to Bengal, and I was therefore totally unprepared to find our steady, sober, and well behaved recruits attacked by disease and die; while the greatest blackguards, those who were always drunk or in the guard-room, possessed comparatively good health. The only way in which this circumstance can be accounted for is, that no weak man can be a drunkard, at least at the age at which recruits generally enter the service, and that our most dissipated men were therefore also the strongest and most capable of resisting disease.

A popular author upon India has said, that disease in that country is not induced by what is drunk so much as by what is eaten; and I am perfectly certain, from my own experience there, that the heavy breakfasts, hot tiffins, rich dinners, and grilled bones at supper, produce more cases of dyspepsia, fever, and dysentery, than all the beer or brandy and water, against both of which we hear so much at home. It is not from either of the latter that so many invalids are annually sent away to the hills, to the Cape, and to England; but it is more frequently to late hours, gambling, and other species of debauchery, that rheumatic affections and worn out constitutions may be traced.

In order to show how the constitution of individuals is affected by their diet, it may be merely stated that the Hindoos, who live almost exclusively upon rice and other vegetable productions, have very little chance of recovering from debilitating diseases, such as cholera. The Mussulmans, on the other hand, who partake of animal food freely, and are not averse to spirituous potations, suffer most from inflammatory diseases; while they bear depletive measures well, and resist the influence of disease of an opposite nature, so much better than the others.

It is well known that in temperate climates less

animal food is required during the summer season than in winter, and that the appetite becomes impaired when the weather is warm, or but little exercise is taken; while a bracing air and active exertion are conducive to it. During the continuance of the hot season in India, very few, even among the youngest and strongest, have much desire for solid food, yet *all* sit down to at least three hot meals daily, at each of which they excite their palate by savory dishes, and when the stomach at last begins to fail, they take an occasional liqueur glassful of brandy with soda water, or a glass of bitter ale, until the evil becomes too great even to be temporarily appeased by such remedies; derangement of the liver is induced, and confirmed dyspepsia destroys all the enjoyments of life.

Among those, however, who lead a more abstemious life, an Indian climate has but comparatively little effect; and the experience of all who have served in that country, proves that disease is best guarded against by avoiding the excessive use of animal food; by taking a moderate quantity of beer, wine, or brandy and water, when feeling exhausted and overcome by the oppressive temperature; by keeping regular hours, and above all by having some mental occupation. Hence it is that civilians in that country are so much more healthy than the military, and that the mortality is greater among bachelors than among the married officers.

It generally happens that persons arriving in the country suffer from a more or less severe attack of fever, attended by derangement of the biliary organs; or from an attack of diarrhæa, within the first few months of their residence. These attacks are generally called *seasoners*, and are supposed to render the individual less liable to the endemic diseases of the country. This however is, I think, very doubtful; for as in England an attack of typhus fever renders the patient more susceptible to another, so it also happens in India, that a person who suffers from one or two attacks within the first year after arriving in the country, may generally be declared a bad subject for India; and, unless speedily removed to his native country, is almost certain to fall a sacrifice to fever in some of its forms; for the disease which may at first be simple-inflammatory, will gradually change its type, and in its future attacks become remittent or intermittent, inducing organic disease of some of the viscera.

Much has been written upon the subject of the seasoning fever, and many eminent authorities have considered that these attacks are naturally beneficial in fortifying the constitution against endemic attacks. In opposition to this opinion, I am inclined to regard the slight inflammatory fever which often occurs on first arriving in India, as a mere consequence of the change of climate and diet, not rendering the person less susceptible to remittent fever, when exposed to the ordinary causes of that disease.

When an European lands in India during the cold season, the system has an opportunity of gradually adapting itself to the climate, as the hot weather comes on; whereas, when he arrives with his *home constitution*, the thermometer at the same time varying from 98° to 102° of Fahrenheit in the house, his system, from not having had an opportunity of accommodating itself to the change, suffers a sudden shock; and as the determination to the liver is always induced by high temperature, an attack of bilious fever, attended by considerable vascular excitement, is the consequence.

When, on the other hand, he lands towards the approach of the rainy season, and happens to be placed in circumstances where he is exposed to malaria, it frequently occurs that if then attacked with fever, it will assume the intermittent or remittent type; it must be borne in mind, however, that a person going to India is not *necessarily* to expect being seized with fever, and that in many instances when they do suffer, the attack can be traced to some act of indiscretion on their own part. And I do not hesitate to assert, that although in many cases we are unable to account for the occurrence of a particular disease, as during an epidemic for instance, still a person may, by accommodating his habits to circumstances, do much to prevent an attack, or to diminish its severity, should he have one.

There is no question, however, that there is *something* in the climate of India peculiarly inimical to the constitutions of Europeans; and that although we occasionally meet with persons who have resided there during half a century and upwards, and who have enjoyed continued good health, still the circumstance, as shown by Dr. Martin,—that there is no instance on record of a *third* generation of pure Europeans who have all been born and resided constantly in the country,—sufficiently proves that India is decidedly destructive to the constitutions of the natives of this country.

CHAPTER II.

REMITTENT FEVER.

Remittent fever — Period and cause — Susceptibility — Symptoms— Morbid appearances—Treatment.

Among the diseases incident to India, the first to claim our attention, is Remittent Fever.

It prevails principally during the latter part of the rainy season, in the months of August and September, when evaporation is rapidly going on, and the noxious vapours arising from decaying vegetable and animal matter, from there often being then little or no wind, float in heavy clouds around our cantonments in the plains. During the prevalence of the disease, there are generally numbers of cases of fever of the intermittent type, particularly tertian and quotidian agues; and it is generally remarked, that the latter, although the simplest form, and most amenable to treatment during its early stages, yet if not speedily checked, is most apt to merge into the remittent; thus shewing that both diseases are mere modifications of each other, differing only in the length of the remissions between the paroxysms.

That some persons are more liable to attacks of fever than others is well known, and can only be accounted for by referring the circumstance to 'peculiarity' of constitution. Thus in India, of two persons who may be equally exposed to miasm, one is soon seized with severe jungle fever, (as it is called); while the other escapes with a slight headache, or perhaps suffers from no indisposition whatever. I am not aware that the drunken and dissipated are more frequently attacked than the steady and sober; but a person after a debauch, when the powers are in a state of exhaustion, is of course in an unfavourable state to resist disease, and therefore, if exposed to the exciting cause of remittent fever, is more apt to be seized, than a person whose vital powers are unimpaired.

The attack may be sudden, or very insidious, and the remissions so indistinct at first, as to readily mislead a person who is unacquainted with the manner in which the disease developes itself. One of the most constant symptoms is headache, a feeling of deep tightness, as if a cord were pulled tight around the brain; the eyebrows are frequently knit from pain, and the eyes suffused.

In all cases then, when a patient is brought to hospital with these symptoms, the medical officer should be prepared to combat a sharp attack, even should they be accompanied by comparatively little pyrexia; for it frequently happens that there is a difficulty at first in distinguishing cases of this disease from those of continued, or of the common intermittent of the country, until the characteristic remission of the symptoms occurs, when of course there can be no more doubt as to the nature of the attack.

During the prevalence of this disease, men are frequently brought to hospital, complaining only of weakness of the lower extremities, and a sensation of coldness in the loins. For a day or two they have felt no inclination for their rations; they have had occasionally dull headaches, with the sight affected by flocculi, and a difficulty of fixing their attention upon any given subject. All this time the surface may be moist, and the pulse not at all affected; but on asking the patient to shew his tongue, it will be observed to be very tremulous and thickly coated with fur; the eyes will be watery and heavy, and a degree of anxiety depicted in the countenance, which could scarcely be expected from the apparently trifling nature of the symptoms. At this period, the administration of an emetic of ipecacuanha, and then a free dose of quinine, as ten grains of the sulphate, in combination with five of extract of hyoscyamus, will sometimes cut the attack short, and always render it much less severe.

The stomach is generally disordered; there is sickness and occasional vomiting of small quantities of bile; while a feeling of listlessness pervades the frame, rendering the patient disinclined to rouse himself to any exertion. When unchecked, these symptoms increase in severity; the headache is, in the early stages of the disease, excruciating; but after a time, from the occurrence of effusion upon the brain, the patient becomes comatose, and, after lingering in that state for a few days, dies with all the symptoms of typhus.

In other cases again, the abdominal viscera suffer. Acute pain is complained of in the intestines; the evacuations are dark, fætid, sometimes streaked with blood, and mixed with vitiated secretions. In such, the symptoms may run into severe dysentery, terminating in extensive ulceration, or sphacelation of the bowels, and death. So that, in the treatment of Remittent Fever, we have in the first place to combat the cerebral affection, and in the second to guard against disease in the intestines. Nor must it be forgotten that the latter complication may be induced by the means employed in the cure; and that a temporary remission of the symptoms, with cool skin and freedom from all pain, very frequently indicates that active disease has attacked the bowels.

When visceral disease is once set in, the patient ceases to have any more of the characteristic remissions and accessions of the fever. In some cases, the inflammation being active, the pulse is for a time increased in strength, the skin becomes hot and dry, and acute local pain is complained of. Such however are not the symptoms from which most danger is to be apprehended; but when we find a sinking of the vital powers, a soft fluttering pulse, dry coated tongue, teeth covered with sordes, sunken glassy eye, and low delirium, a fatal termination must be apprehended.

The surface assumes a peculiar waxy, yellowish tinge, and emits a heavy disagreeable odour; these, with the frequent vomitings of bilious matter show the liver to be much disordered. Digestion is, from the onset of the disease, impaired; there is a loathing of food, and not unfrequently diarrhæa comes on; the stools consisting of little else than dark unhealthy bile, of so acrid a nature as to excoriate the orifice of the rectum. In other instances, however, the patients complain of constipation of several days' duration; and it is generally in these that we have most acute cerebral symptoms.

During my experience of remittent fever in Bengal, I have never met with an instance of the *black vomit,* which is described as the characteristic symptom of a similar disease in the West Indies; but with that exception have seen many die in a state exactly resembling that described by writers upon the latter disease. I have also seen cases of this disease exhibiting as genuine symptoms of typhus as could be met with at home; and were it not for a few remissions at the onset of the attack, they could not be distinguished from it. I am perfectly aware that this statement is in opposition to the opinions of many who have had great experience; for I have frequently heard it asserted that "there was no such disease as typhus in India." It may therefore have been, that in those cases which I met, the typhoid symptoms were merely indicative of extensive disorganization then going on in the intestines; but whether such a thing as idiopathic fever exists, is a question which it is not the object of this paper to examine.

When remittent fever makes its appearance in a regiment, so many cases generally occur in succession, that the disease might not unnaturally be supposed to be propagated by infection; but I am not aware of any practitioner in India who, after a short residence in the country, considers any of its fevers infectious. The circumstances to which its appearance is attributable, affect all in the locality similarly, and hence it is that we have the disease only in low marshy places, or during the rainy season. On examining the bodies of such as die of this disease, we invariably find traces of inflammation in the head, or abdomen, or both. In the former we have effusion upon and within the brain, the arachnoid is in many parts thickened and opaque, the vessels of the membranes congested, on cutting into the substance of the brain, the cut surfaces of vessels appear in vast numbers; and on removing the cerebral mass there is generally a profuse flow of fluid from the base of the skull, and orifice of the spinal canal. In the abdomen we sometimes find redness of different parts of the peritoneum, with occasional adhesions of that membrane. The interior of the small and large intestines may be ulcerated, softened; and in many cases that of the colon is found to be black and sphacelated, while the contents of the gut consist of nothing but a dark fetid fluid. The liver when cut into is generally found gorged with blood, and the gall bladder frequently distended with thick ropy bile. The spleen is found enlarged and softened, particularly where the person had previously been subject to attacks of intermittent fever; but in cases of remittent fever proving fatal, in persons but lately arrived in the country, that organ frequently appears perfectly natural in size and substance.

From what has been said, it will easily be seen that great management is required in the treatment, and that no one method of cure can be applicable to all cases; therefore it is, that before prescribing at all, it is the duty of the medical man to consider carefully what set of organs are most likely to be principally affected, and modify his treatment accordingly.

Venesection, the great sheet anchor in the early stages of almost all fevers, has been found a remedy of very doubtful efficacy in this disease; and it is remarkable how badly it is borne even by plethoric patients. Fainting is generally brought on by the loss of a very few ounces of blood, and the debility induced is very great; the employment of the lancet, therefore, is, as a general rule, to be deprecated in the treatment of remittent fever; for while the relief procured by it is inconsiderable and transient, it invariably renders the convalescence of the patient protracted.

Local bleeding by means of leeches is, however, always attended with benefit; when the patient complains of severe headache, leeches to the temples and cold applications to the scalp, are invaluable remedies; while abdominal symptoms are relieved in a similar way, by leeches and fomentations.

Emetics.—Where there is irritability of the stomach, with bilious vomiting, a dry hot skin, and intense headache, an emetic of simple ipecacuanha is of the utmost benefit; it not only clears the stomach immediately, and empties the gall ducts, but also generally acts as a purge, and unloads the *primæ viæ;* bringing about a temporary remission of the symptoms, during which large doses of calomel and quinine, the main remedies upon which we depend, ought to be administered.

Although emetics are invaluable remedies when properly employed, their use is nevertheless attended by much danger. They ought usually to consist merely of some vegetable production, and I believe none to be so generally applicable as ipecacuanha. They should also be administered in small doses at a time, and repeated every few minutes until their effect be produced. In this way we can generally regulate their action, whereas, when given in one large dose, the excessive vomiting is apt to terminate in cholera, and carry off the patient; and, for a like reason, antimonials must be very carefully employed, when administered at all.

Purgatives.—When the patient complains of constipated bowels, with severe pain in the abdomen; while leeches and fomentations are being applied externally, a pill, containing one to two drops of croton oil with five grains of hyoscyamus, will generally be followed by a free evacuation and relief. When, on the other hand, there is a bilious diarrhœa; a scruple of calomel, with a drachm of tincture of opium, followed in the course of an hour by an ounce of castor oil, will act as a sedative, and for a time procure an interval of rest to the patient, by evacuating the biliary ducts and clearing the bowels of the irritating matter they contained.

Antimonials.—These are remedies which must be employed with great caution, but when well managed are exceedingly serviceable in moderating the violence of the febrile symptoms, so as to procure a short apyrexial period in which other medicines may be advantageously administered. Solution of tartrate of antimony, or antimonial wine, are the best forms in which the medicine can be given; they should be administered in such doses that the patient may take half a grain of the tartrate every half hour, until nausea and slight vomiting are brought about; when a remission generally follows.

Cold affusion is a remedy of the utmost service;

not only in diminishing the temperature of the body directly, but by opening the cutaneous pores, restoring the secretion from the surface, and soothing the patient; so that after days and nights of restlessness, after sponging the body rapidly with water—or what is still better, brandy and water—an interval of comparative ease is experienced, and a sound refreshing sleep induced.

Calomel and Quinine.—These two remedies are spoken of together, as being the sheet anchor in the treatment of remittent fever in the East Indies. During the febrile accessions, a large dose of calomel (as a scruple or twenty-five grains) by acting as a sedative, generally subdues in some measure any urgent symptoms that may be present; and in all cases, when we have reason to suspect that effusion is likely to take place within the head, calomel is the only remedy upon which we can ground any hopes of preventing that termination. It is only during the remission, however, that we can administer calomel in combination with quinine; and therefore it will be well to commence by giving a full dose, as a scruple of calomel, ten grains of sulphate of quinine, and five of extract of hyoscyamus; and following this up by five grains of quinine in solution every half hour, until either the occurrence of nausea, or increase of the headache, warns us to desist, or an accession of the fever comes on. When the state of the bowels is neglected, we must expect that such large doses of powerful medicines will affect the abdominal viscera in some degree; and therefore we need not be surprised on finding, after death in such cases, that the large intestine is filled with unhealthy matter, its interior softened or even sphacelated, and marks of inflammation extensively diffused over both the exterior and interior of the small intestines. To prevent this, it is evident that occasional laxatives are imperatively called for; and I believe the one most generally applicable is a combination of six drachms of castor oil, one drop of croton oil, and thirty drops of tincture of hyoscyamus; which may be given once every day, or every second day, according to circumstances.

The efficacy of calomel in the cure of remittent fever, has been questioned by some medical men in India, who consider that salivation being brought on is merely an indication of the case being likely to terminate favourably; and they say, with truth, that in the greater number of fatal cases in which calomel has been given, the remedy had failed to produce salivation. That is very true; but I am inclined to think that calomel has more virtue as a curative means, than those authors are disposed to allow. But when the medicine is not given early; or, when administered, is combined with immense doses of such a powerful remedy as sulphate of quinine, and when dose after dose is given while the patient is in a state approaching collapse—the bowels having been neglected for days, during which time the practitioner has been relying solely upon calomel and quinine;—the interior of the bowels is then in such a state of disease, that the calomel has no other effect than to increase the disorganisation which most probably had commenced before the remedy was given at all; while a single ounce of castor oil might have prevented it.

In works upon the diseases of India, we are invariably cautioned not to administer quinine when we find the patient's tongue furred; but I fear that were we to follow such instructions implicitly, we should meet with but few cases of remittent or intermittent fever, in which we should consider ourselves justified in employing this invaluable remedy.

During the accessions of fever the tongue is invariably dry, and continues so in very severe cases, even after a remission has taken place. Its surface is then covered with a thick brown fur, which generally is transversely fissured, and principally confined to the centre; the sides and tip being more slightly coated. There is another class of cases in which the tongue becomes as dry as a board, and even fissured, but there is not the smallest particle of fur upon it; on the contrary, the surface is glassy, and very red. In either of these instances, quinine is decidedly inadmissible. Should these indications be accompanied with abdominal symptoms, such as tenderness on pressure, tumefaction, and a dry harsh state of the skin over the epigastrium, and should the alvine evacuations be dark, fetid, and acrid, a dose of castor oil and tincture of hyoscyamus must be immediately administered, leeches applied where most tenderness is felt, and the abdomen afterwards freely fomented; or it may be considered more advisable to administer an enema of castor oil, turpentine, tincture of hyoscyamus, and congee water.

When, on the contrary, the abdominal viscera do not appear to be affected in this way, but the principal determination is to the head; while leeches, cold applications, or blisters are being applied locally, a large dose of calomel will generally have the effect of bringing down the remaining febrile action, and will be speedily followed by the return of a moist state of the tongue as well as of the whole surface. In the most simple cases of remittent and intermittent fevers in India, there is always more or less fur upon the tongue; yet, unless in such instances as those to which we have just alluded, that symptom alone, as already stated, is not considered to contra-indicate the employment of quinine; and I would here remark, that when not given in combination with calomel, its effects will be increased by being mixed with about an equal quantity of powdered rhubarb; in addition to which, the natives, who are very fond of stealing the medicine, will not recognise it when thus disguised, or if they do, it can not be disposed of in the bazaar.

In my opinion, there is only one circumstance which can justify the medical practitioner in India in rejecting the use of calomel in remittent fever, and that is, *disease of the spleen;* it being well known that in cases where that organ is affected, mercury is peculiarly apt to produce the most prejudicial effects, such as phagedemic ulcers, exfoliation of the alveolar portion of the jaws, or even fatal disease of the bowels. It certainly would seem that this viscus has some influence in the generation or purification of the blood; for all subjects in whom it is deranged have a peculiarly sallow and unhealthy appearance, which can never be mistaken, and which gradually disappears as the viscus becomes restored to its normal state; the circumstance of there being no excretory duct, as in other glands, and the very vascular nature of the organ, would also strengthen the inference that it had some specific influence upon the blood, notwithstanding that physiologists have hitherto been unable to ascertain what its precise functions are.

When the symptoms in remittent fever do not yield to the remedies now recommended, and the vital powers begin to sink, diffusible stimuli must of course be employed. In many cases of this disease we find the patient gets into a restless wakeful state, in which he sometimes passes several days and nights; the consequence of which is, that the nervous system becomes affected, and low delirium sets in. Some nicety therefore is required to distinguish such symptoms from the effects of inflammatory action of the brain; for while the latter would demand the employment of antiphlogistic remedies, those now under consideration will be most benefited by a powerful opiate, or a small quantity of some diffusible stimulus, such as wine or beer. Should there be a tendency to coma, a blister must be applied to the nape of the neck; or what is better still, over the whole scalp. When again the abdomen is hot, and harshly dry; when there is tenderness on pressure if made with the tips of the fingers, and the stools are dark and fetid; an enema, consisting of castor oil, turpentine, and rice gruel, must be administered, or a drop or two of croton oil, with five grains of extract of hyoscyamus, given by the mouth.

Such is a very brief account of the remedial means at present employed in the treatment of Remittent, or Jungle Fever, as it occurs in Bengal; but the disease may arise under so many different circumstances, that the treatment must of course be modified accordingly; yet when we see the fearful mortality attendant upon it in that country, we must come to the melancholy conclusion, that however active and scientific our treatment may be, success is but too seldom the recompence of our exertions.

CHAPTER III.

DYSENTERY.

Dysentery — Character — Period and causes — Bad water — Good spirits, a preventive—Wet and Cold—Constipation—Seat of the Disease—Symptoms—Treatment—Results of treatment and remarkable variation —Chronic form—Symptoms—Treatment.

It is but rarely indeed that we meet with a person who has been a few years in India, and has not at some period suffered from this affection in a more or less severe form.

In the medical periodicals of the country we frequently see the question discussed, whether dysentery is inflammatory in its nature, or a disease arising from debility. In whichever of these lights it is viewed, it is, I think, sufficient for the practical physician to know that the remedies most successfully employed in its treatment are those upon which we rely in the cure of inflammation in other parts of the body, whether situated externally or affecting internal organs; only much modified, of course, in consequence of the nature of the viscera in which dysentery is seated.

This disease frequently appears in military stations as an epidemic; and like remittent fever, prevails chiefly towards the latter end of the rainy season; being attributable in no small degree to the impaired quality of the water at this period. That which is obtained from wells and tanks is frequently impregnated with nitre, which abounds in the soil of Bengal; and in addition, contains both animal and vegetable remains in great abundance.

In all barracks, means are provided for filtering and otherwise purifying the water used by the troops, but on a march, where men, as is too frequently the case, are driven to satisfy their thirst by drinking stagnant water from pools on the road sides, it is impossible to prevent the disease. In such cases, one of the best prophylactics is the employment of small quantities of good spirits either *neat*, or, mixed with water. It is almost unnecessary to recommend this to military or civil officers in India; for few are in the country long, before they learn to mix the water with perhaps a little more brandy than is absolutely necessary. Water is, however, seldom used as a beverage; the ordinary drink in the country being beer or soda water.

Bowel affections are also very readily induced by wet and cold, to both of which soldiers are frequently exposed, either in the performances of their military duties, or by their own indiscretion.

Another very fertile cause of dysentery in India is *constipation.* The state of the bowels being neglected, the patient may have only one alvine evacuation in two days, or perhaps not even so often; the general health for some time does not appear to suffer, and therefore no attention is paid to the circumstance. The abdomen becomes slightly tumefied, and it is no uncommon occurrence to hear a person so affected congratulate himself on becoming stout; while in reality he owes his increased corpulency to no other cause than accumulation of hardened fæces in the colon. Sooner or later, the state of the bowels becomes irregular; there is occasional diarrhœa; and in a liquid evacuation there are a greater or smaller number of hardened fæcal masses. There is also slight straining, and a feeling of rawness in the abdomen, which is frequently relieved for a time by a nip of brandy; or the patient may take a dose of castor oil, and for a short time afterwards feel pretty well; but at last the accumulated matter acting as a foreign body, induces irritation, and dysentery is the consequence.

The seat of this disease may, I think, be said to be the mucous membrane and submucous cellular tissue of the large intestine, the morbid action seldom extending upwards beyond the ilio-cælic valve; although in some instances the ilium may also be found to partake of the disease for more than a foot or two from its termination. The ulcers seldom extend through the muscular coat of the intestine; although in some very severe cases, the whole thickness of the gut, particularly about the rectum, may be found destroyed.

The liver is frequently more or less affected in cases of dysentery; but by no means so invariably as some writers would have us believe; for although we may have hepatitis in any of its stages as a complication of dysentery, we find in many post-mortem examinations of the bodies of such men as have died of that affection, that the liver is to all appearances healthy.

One of the earliest and most invariable symptoms of dysentery, is increased secretion of mucus from the lining membrane of the intestine; the stools often consist almost entirely of mucus or slime, also containing blood in greater or less quantity; the calls to stool are frequent and irresistible, the evacuations are unsatisfactory, and the patient complains of a sensation as if some round hard object were lodged in the lower part of the abdomen, for the expulsion of which he makes long and powerful efforts, the violence of the straining being such as, in very severe forms of the disease, to produce prolapsus of a portion of the rectum. The feeling of rawness in the interior of the abdomen increases as the disease advances, until pressure cannot be borne over the epigastrium. The secretion of bile is often increased, occasioning vomiting and continued nausea, or increasing the pain at stool, and causing even excoriation around the anus, by its acrid and vitiated properties.

The surface becomes harshly dry, and a peculiar odour is perceptible, which is so characteristic that an experienced person can distinguish a case of dysentery by it alone. This odour is partly occasioned by the alvine evacuations; it being quite impossible, notwithstanding the greatest attention to personal cleanliness, to prevent small quantities from remaining upon the patient's body or bed-clothes.

The tongue is generally covered with a thick greyish fur; there is much thirst, the patient having a great desire for cold drinks, which invariably increase or induce the irritability of stomach and abdominal pain, while at the same time the calls to stool become more frequent and painful.

The infectious or non-infectious character of dysentery, is a subject which has been duly canvassed by the medical officers who served during the early part of the present century; and, like many other questions, perhaps after all left undecided. As the disease usually occurs in India, it is most assuredly not infectious; but we must remember, in that country the wards of the hospitals are large, well ventilated, and the accommodation for the sick so ample, that they are seldom, if ever, over crowded. The number of servants allowed by the Company is quite sufficient to keep the places clean, and the sick are allowed every possible comfort. The air they breathe is thus never much contaminated; and consequently diseases in which the secretions are affected, are seen in a very different aspect from what they present in crowded and imperfectly ventilated houses and ships. Although we cannot account for the circumstance, we know that the effluvia, arising from a patient labouring under typhus fever, gives rise to a similar disease; it is therefore highly probable that dysentery may in a like manner, under certain circumstances, become capable of being propagated in the same way.

I will venture to assert, that in the treatment of no disease is so much harm done by young medical men lately arrived in India, as in dysentery. It must always be borne in mind, that the diseases of that country run their course far more rapidly, and have less tendency "to work their own cure," than those of Britain, and therefore active and decisive treatment is to be recommended in all cases; nor must we forget that doses of medicine which would in England be considered very large, are but insignificant when employed in the treatment of the diseases of India.

When we find dysentery occurring in a young plethoric person, who has but lately arrived in the country, or who has since his arrival enjoyed good health, we should have no hesitation in abstracting blood from the arm, and continuing the depletion unti lan effect be made upon the system; after which a number of leeches, varying from one dozen to three dozen, or even more, should be applied to the abdomen, and followed by fomentations. In a delicate person, on the other hand, or in a person whose constitution is impaired by dissipation, we must be careful to what extent we abstract blood generally, and therefore leeches alone may be sufficient. When the person has not been attacked with the disease while under the influence of mercury, much benefit will be derived from a large dose of calomel with opium, followed in the course of an hour or two by an ounce of castor oil; or when scybalæ can be detected, a drachm of compound jalap powder. Although calomel, however, is a very excellent remedy, and particularly useful in clearing the gall ducts and improving the secretions, yet it will not of itself cure dysentery, as many persons would seem to imagine, from their almost exclusive employment of it, we therefore cannot too implicitly follow Dr. Johnstone's recommendations, and in the treatment of this disease "endeavour to improve the state of the secretions of the liver and skin."

The effect which ipecacuanha has in severe cases of dysentery, is very remarkable; and although, like every other medicinal agent, apt to fail in particular instances, still as a general rule it ought to be exhibited in combination with hyoscyamus, as soon as possible after the bowels have been well cleared by a dose of laxative medicine. Five grains of ipecacuanha, with an equal quantity of extract of hyoscyamus, should be given every three hours, if such doses can be borne by the patient; but in the event of their occasioning vomiting or severe nausea, the ipecacuanha must be diminished to two or three grains, or altogether omitted; in which case James's powder will be found to be its best substitute.

When there is much pain in the lower part of the abdomen, or the patient complains of the symptom already described as that of a ball in the rectum, an emollient enema may be administered with advantage; and the French method of applying leeches around the anus will in this case materially tend to relieve tormina and tenesmus, by directly unloading the hæmorrhoidal vessels.

Fomentations to the abdomen tend very materially to relieve the pain and subdue the inflammation of the intestines; and therefore ought to be employed as frequently, and for as long a time on each occasion, as possible. In acute attacks of dysentery it is, I think, not advisable to employ counter irritation to the abdomen, such as the application of blisters, or tartar emetic ointment; as by so doing we debar ourselves from the employment of what are generally considered more useful remedies, namely, leeches and fomentations.

Should the pain in the abdomen be relieved by these remedies, and the calls to stool become less frequent, we may conclude that the violence of the attack is abating; but should this favorable change not take place, after having given a fair trial to the usual remedies — viz. general and local bleeding, evacuating the bowels by calomel, followed by castor oil, emollient enemata, and ipecacuanha, in combination with hyoscyamus—another large dose of calomel with opium, succeeded by smaller ones at short intervals, until the pain be relieved, or the mouth become affected, will often produce a favorable change in the symptoms; after which a free dose of some mild laxative should be given, and the ipecacuanha and hyoscyamus again resorted to; it being, however, always borne in mind as a general rule, that the less calomel is given, the more rapid and complete will be the recovery of the patient.

In every case of dysentery, it is necessary to examine the abdomen most carefully, as scybalæ may exist in the cæcum, or other parts of the large intestine; and, by keeping up constant irritation, render the best directed treatment ineffectual. Should they be detected, the employment of laxatives must be persevered in until they shall have been evacuated.

The medical man who has but lately arrived in India, will no doubt be surprised to see such a violent purgative medicine as jalap recommended in the cure of dysentery, in which he may consider that his best endeavours ought to be used for the suppression of the frequent calls to stool; that being one of the most harassing and painful symptoms of which the patient complains. Yet he must guard against being deceived by mere symptoms; for however frequently attempts may be made to evacuate the bowels, it is seldom that more than a little mucus or blood is passed; while it is almost incredible how large a quantity of vitiated secretions and hardened fæces will be brought away, by a free dose of compound jalap powder. We must therefore not be afraid to use it freely; and even should one dose not have the effect of bringing away fæcal matter, a second, and a third dose must be given when the presence of scybalæ is detected; and there are few cases of dysentery in India that have not been preceded by neglect of the bowels.

When the disease has once been checked, the after treatment is very simple; all that is required being to keep the bowels gently open with castor oil, and improve the secretions by giving an occasional dose of blue pill; some bitter, such as gentian or cheryita, being also given two or three times a day, and the patient's diet carefully regulated.

Such is a short sketch of the treatment of dysentery which was pursued in our regimental hospital in India; and as a proof of its success I may mention, that our ratio of deaths from that disease was *one* in *sixty-two admissions*. We found, however, that calomel and opium were more necessary in the upper provinces of Bengal than in the lower; while ipecacuanha and hyoscyamus were more beneficial again in the latter. I frankly confess that I know not how to account for this fact; but my object in writing these observations, is merely to give a plain statement of what I have myself seen during a short service in the East; and in so doing, to confine myself to what occurred within the walls of our own hospital, without attempting to theorise.

I have now to mention a species of dysentery which attacks in a more insidious—and, I would say, a more surely fatal—manner than that which I have already attempted briefly to describe. It occurs among those who have served long in the country, and whose abdominal viscera may therefore be supposed to have been impaired by former disease, or a long course of irregular living superadded to the debilitating effects of an Indian climate.

In it there is no acute pain, no pyrexia; but the patient complains of looseness of the bowels, and describes his stools as of a dark unnatural colour, and very fœtid odour. He suffers much from weakness, and invariably says that he has a feeling of emptiness in the abdomen. His surface is natural, or covered with a clammy perspiration. He speedily takes to his bed; the debility increases, the evacuations continue frequent, and are now attended by some degree of straining, but not much *tormina;* there is intense thirst; acute pain in the abdomen sometimes comes on; in all cases hiccup supervenes; delirium of the low muttering kind comes on, and the patient sinks and dies.

On opening the body in such a case, we find the interior of the large intestine presenting a gangrenous appearance; the mucous membrane much thickened and softened; the disease in some instances extending through the whole thickness of the gut.

I am inclined to think that this form of the disease most frequently affects persons in the better walk of life; and from my experience in it, I fear medical treatment is at best but palliative.

When a primary attack of acute dysentery has not been effectually cured, or the patient has suffered from repeated attacks, the disease generally terminates in the CHRONIC FORM, from which he has very little chance of recovery while he remains in the country. Hence it is that so many private soldiers annually die of it; for while it is always comparatively easy to send officers to sea or to the hills, there are very few opportunities of sending the men away while they are capable of benefiting by change of climate.

There is such a variety in the symptoms which attend chronic dysentery, that it is almost impossible to give a minute description of them. In all cases, however, they are sufficiently distinct to point out the real nature of the case even to the most inexperienced. There is, as might be expected, much emaciation; the abdomen is sunken; the anterior parietes retracted towards the spine: there is more or less tenderness upon pressure, and a gurgling noise in different parts as the hand is moved along the course of the large intestine. The evacuations are frequent, unsatisfactory; and although attended by less pain than in the acute form, nevertheless occasion the patient much suffering. The stools vary much in colour and consistence, being seldom the same for two days in succession. At one time they are pale, and devoid of bile, at another green, or even black; sometimes streaked with blood, at others containing clots, but always mixed with large quantities of mucus.

In the treatment of such cases, we must keep two objects in view; to improve the state of the secretions, and support the strength of the patient. The first of these we endeavour to do by alteratives and astringents, the second by tonics and regimen. In all cases of chronic dysentery we may conclude that there is ulceration present in some part of the large intestine; we ought therefore to allow the vitiated secretions to remain as short a time as possible, as by removing them, one cause of irritation is taken away, and a chance given to nature of working her own cure.

Small doses of castor oil ought therefore to be given occasionally, and we shall find it of great advantage to administer it in combination with some vegetable astringent and tonic. A draught of two or three drachms of oil, two drachms of tincture of rhubarb, and one of compound tincture of gentian, may be repeated once every twenty-four hours; and if mixed with a little warm coffee, its unpleasant flavour will scarcely be perceived. An occasional small dose of blue pill, or hydrargyrus cum creta, will be found useful in stimulating and evacuating the liver. Ipecacuanha and hyoscyamus may also be employed advantageously, when the increase of pain and tenesmus denote a slight accession of inflammation; in which case it may likewise be necessary to apply a few leeches and fomentations, or to administer an emolient enema. The moderate use of animal food, together with port wine, is generally necessary.

Various mineral astringents have been recommended from time to time, the principal of which are sulphates of copper, iron, and zinc—nitrate of silver, and acetate of lead,—all of which have been employed with various success. We must bear in mind, however, that no one remedy can be applicable in all cases, even of the same disease; and as sure as we make a hobby of any single remedy, to the exclusion of others, so surely must the lives of our patients be in jeopardy. It is therefore our duty, when we find one method of treatment fail, to try another ; yet of course without running to the opposite extreme of pusillanimity and indecision in our practice.

CHAPTER IV.

HEPATITIS.

Hepatitis—Cause—Effect of Beer and Spirits—Heavy meals and inactivity—Native habits—Symptoms—Treatment—Peculiar effect of Mercury—Exploring the Liver.

It is said that about one in every six Europeans who die in India, is carried off by Hepatitis, either in its acute or chronic form; hence this disease may be regarded as being in the East what pulmonary consumption is in Britain. The heat of an Indian climate must doubtless be looked upon as one of its most constant, predisposing, as well as exciting causes; but the mode of life generally followed by residents in that country, has also a very material influence upon the functions of the liver.

I do believe that wine or beer—nay, brandy and water, in moderation—are necessary in India to counteract the debilitating effects upon the constitution of a hot season in the plains. Either of these, however, when employed too frequently, or in too large quantities, must speedily affect the liver; while the habit of eating heavy meals during the heat of the day, and then after a meal of hot animal food taking a sleep for several hours, will sooner or later give rise to congestion of that organ. It would be well for us, were we to modify our habits according to the climate in which we live, and adopt some hints which the natives from generation to generation have learned from nature. They never eat in the middle of the day, when it can possibly be avoided; and those who indulge in animal food take much less during the hot, than in the cold season of the year. Their chief food in summer consists of pulpy and cooling fruits; while they pay scrupulous attention to the state of the bowels; one or all of these points being constantly neglected by Europeans in that country.

It is not a point of much consequence *in practice* to know what set of vessels are principally affected in hepatitis, yet some authors have amused themselves by attempting to trace the disease to one particular class; some referring it to the ramifications of the hepatic artery, and others to the vena porta. The very circumstances, however, of so much discussion having taken place upon the subject, proves how difficult it is to refer it exclusively to one.

"Liver" may occur unconnected with any other disease, or be present in cases of fevers of the intermittent or remittent type, or of dysentery; in all of which it is a most important complication. Its peculiar tendency is speedily to run on to suppuration; pus being apparently formed with greater rapidity in this organ, than in any other. It is not in those cases where there is most acute pain or pyrexia, that we most dread this unfavorable termination; but it is in those where there is a dull heavy pain deeply seated in the side, with comparatively little disturbance of the system, that we have most to fear the occurrence of abscess; these being the symptoms which distinguish inflammation of the parenchyma of the liver, from that of its peritoneal coverings; which, although the most painful, is by far the least dangerous of the two forms of this disease.

There may occasionally be considerable difficulty in distinguishing inflammation of the liver from pneumonia. Percussion and auscultation may certainly render the diagnosis easy in the early stages of the disease; but in cases of long standing, the liver, from enlarging upwards, presses upon the lower lobe of the right lung, thus giving rise to symptoms which may altogether mask the primary disease. When however the organ attains such a size, as to encroach permanently upon the thoracic cavity, disease speedily attacks the lung; terminating in hepatisation, or in pulmonary abscess.

Those who have seen much of acute hepatitis in a hot climate, soon become alive to the fact, that in all cases, active measures must be employed; and that they are equally necessary when the pain is dull but deep, with little alteration in the pulse, as when the symptoms are more distinct. It is a pity that medical men should attempt to draw such a wide distinction between congestion and inflammation of the liver; for as in both there is superabundance of blood in the organ, impeding the performance of its functions, there can be less harm done by treating a case actively from the outset, than by trifling with remedies which at best but relieve the symptoms for a little, without subduing the disease.

In the treatment, loss of blood is the first grand step to be taken, and this can be effected by opening a vein, or by applying leeches, or by both, according to the age, strength, and habits of the patient. After that, a free dose of calomel must be given, and followed in the course of an hour or two by a sharp purge; than which, I believe, none can be better than the compound extract of colocynth, or compound powder of jalap. Emetics are frequently recommended, and are, without doubt, very valuable remedies; yet I think it would be better to clear the *prima via*, by means of a cathartic, than to administer an emetic, the action of which must increase the patient's sufferings. In all cases, our object ought to be to bring the system under the influence of mercury as speedily as possible; therefore, after the employment of the above measures, calomel must be given in free and often repeated doses.

Some authors affect to doubt the superior efficacy of mercury in hepatitis; and among others a late writer on the diseases of India, who says, "What, it may be asked, does calomel possess which renders it superior to croton oil, opium, and tartar emetic, the three representatives of these classes of medicines?" In reply to this query, it may be said that it possesses a remarkable power of preventing suppuration, which neither of these remedies does; and is, in consequence, peculiarly applicable to the treatment of hepatitis, whose tendency, as every one knows, is to run rapidly on to the formation of abscess.

When hepatitis occurs in a young and otherwise healthy subject, it is, generally speaking, by no means an intractable disease; the acute symptoms in the vast majority of cases being readily subdued by the remedies already mentioned; and the cure completed by the continued employment of purges, counter irritation to the side, and abstemious diet. When, however, the inflammation runs on to suppuration, a less favourable issue of the case is to be apprehended; and then our first object is the removal of the patient to a cold climate, when such a step is practicable.

The occurrence of suppuration in the liver is indicated by a very distinct rigor, succeeded by hectic flushes and diarrhæa, which exhaust the strength of the patient: or death may ensue from the abscess evacuating itself into the lungs, and producing suffocation, or causing fatal peritonitis, by opening into the cavity of the abdomen.

In such cases, when there is one large abscess in the substance of the liver, death must soon ensue; but when there are one or more small ones, I believe a person may prolong his days, and enjoy comparative comfort, by returning to Europe, and by careful attention to diet and regimen. The slightest excess at table, however, or imprudent exposure to the weather, will almost to a certainty occasion an acute attack; the occasional recurrence of which so undermines the constitution, that it will at last sink under the disease.

The most useful remedies in the treatment of

chronic hepatitis may be briefly stated to consist of laxatives, containing blue pill or calomel, counter irritation to the side, the nitro-muriatic-acid bath; and diluted nitric acid internally, which seems to have some specific action upon the liver, serving to restore its tone after an attack of inflammation. We are at a loss how to account for this peculiar effect; but it is equally puzzling to describe the action of any other remedial agent; unless indeed, like some modern authors, we attribute it all to *electricity*. It is sufficient for practical purposes, however, to know that certain remedies have particular effects; and if we use that knowledge aright in the treatment of disease, it is all that can be reasonably required of us.

A few years ago, the practice of *exploring* the liver for abscesses, and evacuating them, when they could be found, by means of a trocar and canula, was very fashionable in India; but like every other antiquated fashion, it has had its day, and fallen into disuse. Of the success of the practice, I am unable to speak from personal experience; but I have examined the bodies of men who had, during life, been *explored* for abscess by physicians of high reputation in their profession, and whose livers after death presented *no trace* of disease; so that it is very evident some blunder must have been committed in the over zeal of the operators. In those cases, however, where the abscess projects under the ribs, common sense will dictate the propriety of making an opening into it; but when there is a doubt as to where the abscess actually is, it must, I think, be looked upon as a measure of very doubtful propriety, to explore the liver in a variety of directions, until the escape of matter shows that a cavity containing pus has been entered; while the injuries inflicted by the instrument must have had the effect of setting up fresh inflammation, of an equally, if not more severe nature than the original disease.

CHAPTER V.

CHOLERA.

Symptoms—Whether Contagious or not—Causes—Variety—Morbid appearances—Treatment—Hydrocyanic Acid—Disuse of Opium—Secondary Fever prevented.

THIS disease carries off more persons in India than perhaps any other, yet its pathology is but very imperfectly understood. Were the question asked, "What is Cholera?" nine-tenths of the medical profession would answer,—and answer correctly,—"I do not know"; while the remaining one-tenth would most probably indulge in some vague speculation, at variance alike with the dictates of common sense, and all the known laws of nature. All we know of the disease is, that it is generally attended by profuse vomiting and purging of a clear liquid, resembling rice water; and from the immense quantities evacuated, we can only account for its generation, by supposing it to be the serum of the blood, of which there is hæmorrhage going on from the inner surface of the stomach and bowels.

The other most prominent symptoms are, suppression of the natural secretions, a rapid sinking of the vital powers, and spasms of the muscles of the extremities and abdomen. So characteristic is the general appearance of a cholera patient, that any person who has once seen a case of the disease, can never forget the sunken eye surrounded by a bluish zone, the contracted features, and the fearful anxiety which is depicted in the expression of the countenance.

The attack usually comes on towards morning, in the form of simple diarrhæa. After two or three fæcal evacuations, the stools assume the characteristic rice-water appearance. There is at first mere irritability of the stomach, which speedily terminates in obstinate vomiting. Spasms occur in different parts of the body and extremities; there is extreme restlessness; and from the earliest stages of the disease the patient has an utter carelessness of life, seeming to look upon death as a welcome deliverer from his sufferings. The thirst is intense; the patient complains of burning heat within him, which makes him crave for cold drinks, and throws off his bedclothes as if that gave him relief; while the tongue, breath, and surface, are deadly cold, and the fingers corrugated, as if they had been for a long time immersed in water. The pulse is exceedingly rapid and small, becoming generally weaker and weaker until its beat at the wrist is imperceptible. The features collapse, the eyes sink, the voice becomes a hoarse whisper, the face and whole surface of the body assume a slate-blue tint; and if these symptoms are not checked, the powers of life begin to sink, the spasms become less severe, vomiting and purging less urgent, the patient appears more calm, he stretches himself in bed, and appears literally to "fall asleep in death."

In the generality of fatal cases, death takes place within twelve hours after the attack; and from what I have seen of the disease, I am inclined to think that in those cases which prove fatal after the second day, death is not so much caused by the disease as by the remedies employed in the treatment; giving rise to cerebral and abdominal affections, constituting what is called *Secondary Fever*.

A very important question arises as to the contagious or non-contagious nature of cholera; and many circumstances would seem to warrant us in including it among the first of these classes of diseases; although, from what I have seen of it, I do not consider that, under ordinary circumstances, it is propagated by personal contact.

Although it occasionally appears sporadically in a regiment, yet it generally occurs as an epidemic; its commencement being attended by nothing remarkable in the state of the atmosphere—the most delicate chemical experiments having failed to detect any difference in the composition of the air on such occasions. After raging for a time with more or less severity, it may disappear as suddenly and as unaccountably as it commenced; or it may proceed in a different direction, ravaging a certain line of country, or taking the course of a particular river.

It is true that those whose duty it is to attend upon cholera cases, are very frequently attacked by the disease; and patients who occupy contiguous beds to that in which there is a case of this disease, may become similarly affected. Yet I do not consider these facts sufficient to prove that cholera is either infectious or contagious; for during an epidemic all are alike exposed to whatever influence produces the disease, and are, in my opinion, equally liable to be attacked, whether they have intercourse with those who are labouring under it or not.

Very few detachments of European troops ever proceed up or down the country by the Ganges, without suffering more or less from cholera; one or two cases only of the disease sometimes occurring, while on other occasions it visits every boat in a fleet, and continues its devastations for weeks together. As a probable cause of its frequency on the river, I may mention that the Ganges for several hundred miles runs in a bed of soft alluvial soil; that during the rains it overflows its banks, inundating the country on each side to an almost incredible extent; as for instance, about Bhangulpore and Monghyr, where, during the summer months, it is scarcely more than a mile in breadth; while during the rainy season it extends to *ten*. As this mass of water decreases, it of course leaves a frightful extent of soil containing a large amount of decaying animal and vegetable matter, from which the most pernicious miasmata arise, occasioning fevers, dysentery, and no doubt cholera also.

Two species of the disease occur in India,—namely, the spasmodic, and the asphyxiated, which is comparatively rare but is by far the most fatal of the two; its only peculiarity is that the spasms of the former are altogether absent, or of very trifling severity, but the prostration of strength is extremely rapid; the vomiting in some cases not very urgent, but the lips and entire surface speedily assume a blue livid appearance, death apparently being occasioned by the mal-oxygenation of the blood.

On examining the bodies of those who have died of cholera, we are struck with the absence of all appearances which, under ordinary circumstances, would account for death. We always find extensive congestion of the venous system, the right side of the heart being gorged with dark liquid blood; and what is a remarkable feature in this disease, is the total absence of those coagula in the heart and large venous trunks, which are usually discovered after death from other diseases. The stomach and bowels are remarkably pale; and their inner surface coated with a soft ropy matter, as if it had been smeared over with very thick mucilage. The stomach usually contains a greater or smaller quantity of the medicines which have been administered in the course of treatment; and the lower part of the intestinal canal is filled with the characteristic rice-water fluid. In so far as the other viscera are concerned, we find nothing that can be said to be connected with this disease in particular, except that the gall bladder is in every case immensely distended with dark ropy bile, and the urinary bladder as invariably contracted and empty.

There is one remarkable circumstance invariably

to be observed in the bodies of those persons who have died of cholera, which is, that while during the last hours of life the surface is deadly cold, the temperature *increases* for some time after dissolution, and continues high for a considerable period. This phenomenon is certainly very peculiar; and, so far as I am aware, has not been satisfactorily explained; yet those who have seen anything at all of Asiatic cholera, know well that it constantly does occur.

In considering the treatment, I may briefly premise, that for years and years medical men seem to have completely thrown aside all the ordinary physiological principles by which the treatment of disease in general is conducted, and have had recourse to remedies the most empirical and unprofessional. Thus, at one time all patients affected with cholera had saline mixtures injected into their veins; while red hot irons were drawn along each side of the spine, from the nape of the neck to the sacrum; their craving thirst being all the time tantalised by giving occasional spoonfuls of *water-gruel*. Then came a system of aggravating the vomiting, which is one of the most painful symptoms of the disease, by giving table spoonsful of powdered mustard; and then, as if that were not sufficient, the sinking energies of life were systematically destroyed by large doses of one of the most powerful depressants in the pharmacopeia, tartar emetic. Epsom salts and croton oil were also employed apparently for the same purpose; and then the patients were taken out of bed to die under a constant inundation of cold water, by having buckets of it thrown over them; an apology for treatment being made by giving three grains of calomel with one of opium; and should the patient survive three hours, *repeating* the *dose*.

Bleeding to a moderate extent was, and is still, considered by many as a remedy of great importance in the treatment of this disease; its modus operandi being, as they suppose, to relieve the over distension of the heart, and, lessening the oppression upon that organ, give a chance to its paralysed fibres to recover their former tone. I do not think, however, that venesection comes up to the expectations of most of its advocates; and, as a remedy, is only useful in the very earliest stages of the disease, when the spasms are very severe, and the patient is of a very full plethoric habit.

Our treatment must of course be modified by the stage of the disease, and the natural constitution of the patient. Thus, for a person within the first half hour after the symptoms have manifested themselves, a glass of brandy may be sufficient to remove the disease and effect a cure; but when the disease has once been regularly established, such simple means will have but little effect, and then it becomes necessary to employ the most active treatment.

If we find the patient suffering from severe spasms, with urgent vomiting and purging, the pulse at the wrist being at the same time tolerably good, our best treatment will be to administer from a scruple to half a drachm of calomel; following it up by a stimulating mixture, composed of spirits of camphor, aromatic spirits of ammonia, and sulphuric ether; the thirst being allayed by cold brandy and water. Should the stomach reject the first dose, another must be immediately administered; but if, after the second or third dose of calomel, the vomiting continue obstinate, five or six drops of the medicinal hydrocyanic acid in a little water, repeated as often as it is rejected, will frequently subdue this symptom when all other means have failed; after which the ordinary remedies are immediately to be had recourse to again. This treatment, I am aware, is novel; but from what I have seen of it, my firm conviction is, that no risk can arise from the largeness of the dose, if due care be paid in desisting from its further employment, after its effects have once manifested themselves; and I feel satisfied that by prussic acid

I have saved the lives of many, in whom the disease would have otherwise proved fatal.

I cannot but regret that I had not an opportunity of giving this medicine a trial upon a more extensive scale, as I feel satisfied that it is one of the utmost value in the treatment of cholera; checking the spasmodic action of the stomach by its sedative powers, when all the means hitherto employed have failed, and producing no tendency to *secondary* disease; which, I have no hesitation in saying, some medicines, as they are at present employed, do.

To the best of my knowledge, I am the first person who has employed prussic acid in the treatment of this disease; and in recommending it, shall no doubt be expected to explain my reasons for giving it such a preference as a remedy calculated to subdue the urgent vomiting in such cases. I therefore beg to remark briefly, that this symptom being unattended by any other which would induce us to refer it to inflammatory irritation of the stomach, we can only attribute it to derangement of the nervous system, upon which prussic acid is well known to act direct as a most powerful sedative.

Calomel is the next most important medicine; acting in the first instance as a sedative, and, secondly, stimulating the gall ducts, which are spasmodically closed. When, however, the disease has existed for several hours before medical treatment has been applied for, and the vital powers have begun to sink—as we soon discover by the imperceptible pulse, the hollow voice, and death-like coldness of the surface—calomel will be found perfectly useless, unless we can revive the energies of life by powerful stimulants by the mouth and in the form of enema; by the employment of frictions to the extremities, and strong blisters or a mustard poultice to the epigastrium.

In the vast majority of such cases, our best endeavours fail to revive a person who has once fallen into the stage of collapse, as this state is called; but when we are so fortunate as to restore a little vital action, so that the pulse can be felt at the wrist or temples, a large dose of calomel should be immediately given; smaller ones, as ten grains, being afterwards repeated every half hour at first, and then less and less frequently, as bile begins to make its appearance in the stools,—the intervals being occupied in the administration of stimulants; and I may here mention, that in these cases, a little port wine in hot sago is frequently relished by the patient, and is of much benefit in allaying the irritability of stomach and nausea, which the constant administration of medicine is very apt to induce.

The favourable symptoms are the re-appearance of the secretions which have been checked, as the occurrence of bile in the stools, the discharge of urine, and the restoration of the natural warmth and moisture of the surface; when these do appear, we must not suddenly desist in our treatment, but are gradually to diminish the dose of our medicines, allowing the intervals between each to become longer and longer; nor must we neglect to keep the bowels open three or four times during the twenty-four hours for the first two or three days of convalescence, for there is at first always a great tendency to constipation. The bile having once made its appearance, flows in such immense abundance, that the evacuations frequently appear to consist of nothing else; which it is also discharged in large quantities from the stomach. Its evacuation must therefore be encouraged, its presence in the intestines being apt to set up disease of the most serious nature. A mild laxative dose must therefore be given at first every morning and evening, but afterwards only once a day. Two or three drachms of castor oil, with some carminative, is as useful as any; but it is very apt to produce nausea and vomiting, in which case two drachms of tincture of rhubarb, with an equal quantity of compound tincture of gentian, will be found to answer every purpose.

We must not allow ourselves to be deceived by the dark appearance which the evacuations frequently assume, after a few doses of calomel have been taken, and which may depend upon the decomposition which takes place between that substance and the sulphurated gases secreted in the intestinal canal; the slightest attention, however, will be sufficient to distinguish such a stool from that coloured by bile.

Should there be any determination to the head or abdomen, it is to be treated by local and general bleeding, and other ordinary means, according to circumstances; and as regards secondary fever, I am of opinion that it only occurs when the free employment of laxatives has been neglected in the early period of the patient's convalescence.

When cholera terminates favourably, the recovery is remarkably rapid; but one attack does not render a person exempt from another, nor does the person who has once had the disease appear to be more liable to it at a future period than any one else. In fact, cholera seems to have no respect for either sex or age; it attacks the sober as well as the dissipated, and those who have been years in the country, as well as the newly arrived.

Some persons may wonder how it is that in the short sketch of cholera which I have just given, I have never so much as mentioned *opium*; my reason is, that I think its efficacy in the treatment of this disease has been much overrated, and my success was much greater after I *excluded* it altogether from the treatment, than it was while I employed it as I had been taught by lecturers and authors. I found that it had but little, if any, effect in checking the more urgent symptoms, such as vomiting, purging, and spasms; and that its free exhibition rendered patients particularly liable to secondary fever, attended with severe cerebral affection.

CHAPTER VI.

APOPLEXY.

Peculiarity—Cause—Influence of inactivity and exercise—Symptoms —Morbid appearances—Treatment.

In considering this disease as it occurs in India, it is to be understood that I particularly allude to what is known in that country under the name of Sun-stroke, or "Apoplexy of the hot winds," from its prevalence at that particular season, and not to that form of the disease which is met with at home, accompanied by sanguineous effusion within the head.

I may venture to say that we are altogether ignorant of the proximate cause of the disease; for in many post mortem examinations we are surprised to find no appearance to account for death. It being then of such a peculiar nature, I shall only briefly describe the symptoms and usual progress of this species of apoplexy, and offer a few remarks upon the treatment which is recommended to be pursued.

Although it usually prevails from the middle of April to the middle of June, when the hot winds are at their height, it does not appear that mere exposure to their direct influence, will of itself produce the disease; for we find it occurring as frequently, if not more so, among those who are much within doors, as among those who appear less careful of themselves. This circumstance would lead us to believe that exercise, even in the very hottest season, is more beneficial to Europeans in India, than the usual habit of lying in a state of inactivity for many hours during the day. In order, too, to show how little this disease is influenced by habits and mode of life, I may mention, that soldiers in solitary confinement, or in hospital, are equally liable to the disease as those in barracks; although in many cases an attack is most assuredly induced by drinking to a large extent, and then lying exposed to the sun, as is too frequently the case among our troops in India.

The attack is in general preceded by no particular premonitory symptom. Sometimes the patient complains of headache; but generally the first indication of the occurrence of the disease is that he appears somewhat stupid, and for a time talks incoherently. It is seldom, however, that there is any particular excitement; but, on the contrary, stupor seems to come on, and gradually increase, until it ends in complete coma. The breathing then becomes stertorous; the pupils in some cases dilated, in others contracted, but in all insensible to the stimulus of light; the lips livid, and frothy mucus issues from the mouth; but the peculiar symptom which at once distinguishes this disease from sanguineous apoplexy, or coma from ordinary compression upon the brain, is the very high temperature which the surface generally acquires, and which is peculiarly intense over the epigastric region. It is not only present from the earliest stages of the disease, but continues for several hours after dissolution. Nor has it escaped the notice of the natives of India; who, in consequence of this symptom, refer the disease to "combustion of the liver," induced by the intense heat of the sun.*

The progress of this disease is more rapid than that of any other with which I am acquainted; death usually occurring in from four to eight hours after the commencement of the attack.

The appearances discovered after death are gene-

* The natives of India consider the liver to be the centre of the circulation of the blood, and also the seat of the softer passions, which in this country are usually said to reside in the heart.

rally unsatisfactory, there being seldom any appreciable increase in the quantity of serum naturally existing in and around the brain. Sometimes, however, there is more, and in such cases the arachnoid membrane presents traces of inflammatory action, it being in some parts thickened and opaque; the substance of the brain will likewise present a larger number of red points than natural, when cut into; and the choroid plexuses will be somewhat congested.

I have never remarked any morbid appearance in the abdomen which can be said to be peculiar to this disease, but have been led to understand that inflammation and gangrene of duodenum have been observed in the bodies of many persons who have died of "sun-stroke." There is much obscurity in the post mortem appearances, and those who have an opportunity should direct their attention to its pathology.

It is a matter of very great difficulty to recommend any particular mode of treatment, where all seem to be alike unsuccessful; as is most assuredly the case in the disease now under consideration.

Bleeding might, à priori, be considered useful; but those who have seen much of this disease know from experience how rapidly death ensues after the employment of the lancet; the patient frequently dying in our hands while performing the operation. Nor do leeches to the temples appear to produce any benefit. Our treatment consisted in giving a large dose of croton oil, with hyoscyamus internally; administering a strong turpentine enema, shaving the head and employing cold affusion freely, afterwards applying a large blister to the scalp; but out of all the cases of this disease which I have seen treated, (between sixty and eighty), in only one did I succeed in restoring the patient to consciousness, but a relapse speedily took place, which terminated in death.

CHAPTER VII.

DELIRIUM TREMENS.

Causes—Symptoms—Post-mortem appearances—Treatment.

I HESITATED before introducing this disease as one of those most prevalent among Europeans in India; but from the frequency with which cases of it occur in our regiments serving in that country, I trust a brief description of the affection will not be considered altogether out of place here.

It is well known that immoderate indulgence in wine gives rise to gout. So, in like manner, delirium tremens is induced by drinking spirits; and really, when we meet with persons in India whose daily allowance is a bottle, or a bottle and a half, of brandy or gin, in addition to their quantum of beer and wine, we no longer feel surprised at the prevalence of this disease among them. The medical man who first joins a regiment there, will not be prepared to find that the subjects of delirium tremens are in many instances old soldiers who possess badges for good conduct, and even non-commissioned officers. But he will soon learn that it is not always those who appear most frequently in the defaulters' book, who are in reality the most dissipated; but that those who really are the greatest drunkards generally possess rather good characters, merely because, in the barrack-room phrase, "they drink at proper times," that is, when they are not likely to be put on duty; and as soldiers have next to nothing to do during the hot season, those who are inclined to excess have numberless opportunities of indulging.

It is impossible to define the quantity of spirits necessary for a person to drink before delirium tremens is induced; but one attack of the disease renders the subject of it more liable to a return, and the severity of the attacks always increases in proportion to the frequency of their recurrence. Hence it is that in young soldiers a cure is generally easily effected; while in the old and dissipated, the disease is always obstinate, and attended with danger.

Those persons who have for years led an irregular and dissipated life, are well known to be less capable of resisting the effects of an injury, than those whose constitutions have not been impaired by such causes; and accordingly symptoms of delirium tremens sometimes manifest themselves when such subjects have met with a severe accident, as a fracture or dislocation. It is doubtful, however, how far the disease in these instances may not have been induced by the treatment to which the patients are subjected in hospital; where they may perhaps have been suddenly deprived of a stimulus which the medical attendant had no means of knowing was habitual to them, and the continuance of which had been rendered doubly necessary by such accident. But my present object is briefly to describe the disease as it occurs after hard drinking, and when it is not complicated with local injury.

In many of its symptoms it closely resembles phrenitis; from which disease it is, however, distinguished by occurring *after* a debauch; whereas phrenitis, when arising from that cause, comes on while the person is indulging. Delirium tremens is characterised from the earliest stages by extreme restlessness on the part of the patient; he moves about in a hurried and excited manner; the mind is at the same time more or less affected—in the slighter forms of the disease, being disturbed regarding some matter connected with his ordinary occupation; there is a constant dread of some fancied impending danger; and in severe cases the hallucinations become of such a frightful character, that the disease has obtained among soldiers the very appropriate name of "The Horrors." He is impressed with the idea that there is some conspiracy formed against his life; and when he is in bed, fancies that he is beset by venomous reptiles, or surrounded by murderers. At last so alarmed does he become at the phantoms which haunt his disturbed imagination, that he falls into a state of despondency for a time; and then the desire of self-destruction is so powerful, that he must be carefully watched, lest he should find means of committing suicide.

The idea that the patient is pursued by the evil spirit, is invariably present in cases of this disease; and I shall never forget one case in which an old soldier was kept in a frightful state of horror for several days and nights by that awful hallucination. The treatment employed for a long time failed to procure relief; but at last he seemed to obtain a little rest, and we began to entertain hopes that the case would terminate favourably; when suddenly he sprang upright in bed, called upon the Hospital Sergeant to save him from the devil, who he said was dragging him away; then uttering a wild shriek he fell back convulsed, and almost instantly expired.

There is in almost every case obstinate constipation of the bowels; the tongue is thickly covered with an ash-grey loose flocculent-looking fur, which is in a very great measure characteristic of this disease, and when protruded is so very tremulous that the patient appears to have lost all power over it; the hands too, and in fact the whole frame, is in a state of constant tremor; the pulse is not generally much affected; the surface is of natural temperature, and covered with a clammy perspiration; and there is very considerable thirst. Although the patient, when left to himself, invariably continues to talk incoherently, still on the approach of the surgeon, he appears to summon all his energies, and for a time will answer questions correctly. The effort by which he collects his wandering ideas is but of brief duration, for within a few minutes he will relapse into his former state.

As in all instances where the mind is affected, there is an extraordinary degree of cunning observable in patients labouring under this disease, who sometimes acquire an unaccountable antipathy to some of their comrades or attendants, and frequently have recourse to most ingenious plans to obtain a favourable opportunity of injuring or murdering the object of their suspicion or hatred. A medical officer must therefore be careful, that when he is near such a person a third party be in the room; as the patient generally tries to obtain possession of a knife or razor, with which he may attempt to commit murder or self-destruction.

Death may be caused by apoplexy, in which case a clot of blood will be discovered on examining the brain; but in the greater number of instances, the post mortem appearances will be mere congestion of the cerebral vessels. There may also be a larger than natural quantity of fluid in the ventricles of the brain, and base of the skull; and in the cases of old drunkards, a distinct odour of spirits is emitted, when an incision is made into the brain, so as to lay open the ventricles. Many persons have questioned the possibility of such a circumstance; and I too had many doubts upon the subject, until I was afforded an opportunity of observing it in more cases than one, which occurred in the regimental hospital at Allahabad.

In all cases of delirium tremens, although the symptoms appear alarming from the very commencement, yet they are not generally so in reality; it being only among old dissipated men, who have suffered from frequent attacks of the disease, that danger is usually to be apprehended. A surgeon, however, who has not been accustomed to treat it, might occasion the most serious consequences, were he to employ the remedies which the character of the symptoms would appear to indicate.

General bleeding is, as a general rule, invariably to be avoided in the treatment of this disease, even when there appears to be the greatest excitement; but when there is very evident determination of blood to the head, as indicated by flushed countenance, suffused eyes, and heat of scalp, a few leeches may be advantageously applied to the temples; although, as these symptoms generally depend upon the confined state of the patient's bowels, they will as generally be relieved by a smart purgative. From the convenient way in which croton oil can be administered, it is particularly eligible in these cases, when, as the patient never considers himself otherwise than in the rudest possible health, he wonders what he has to do with medicine. A little coaxing, however, will induce him to swallow a lump of sugar; and with it two, or even three, drops of croton oil.

After having freely evacuated the bowels, our next object is to procure sleep, to which end all our endeavours must be directed. Opium is the main remedy on which we ought to rely, and it will be well to commence by giving a couple of drachms of the tincture, in a pint of porter, if that is to be procured, or if not, in an equal quantity of beer; and follow this up with five grains of the country hill-opium every hour; varying it three times during the day, by substituting the dose of laudanum and beer. These doses are no doubt large, but the Indian opium is considerably weaker than that with which we are supplied in this country; and if administered in smaller quantities, it might only produce the stimulating effect of the drug, instead of acting as a soporific. I have myself administered upwards of half an ounce of the hill opium in an obstinate case of delirium tremens, before I succeeded in inducing sleep, and with perfect success; hence I consider there is little danger to be apprehended from the largeness of the quantity of the drug which is given, provided it be administered as I have recommended, and care at the same time be taken that the patient's bowels be moved once or twice in the twenty-four hours.

Should the case prove obstinate, a blister must be applied to the scalp; or what appears preferable, to the back of the neck; and after it has produced free vesication, the raw surface is to be dressed with a little simple dressing, upon which a few grains of powdered opium have been sprinkled. In fact, every possible means of introducing the medicine into the system ought to be had recourse to; and as it is necessary to continue the artificial stimulus in which the patient had been indulging prior to the attack, he ought to have two or three pints of beer or porter daily at least, as well as one or two glasses of spirits. His thirst will be best relieved by a little lime juice and water, or an occasional effervescing draught; and should he complain of hunger, he may have a mutton chop well seasoned with pepper.

The mental hallucinations of the patient must also be carefully attended to. When he has an idea that his bed is infested with reptiles, or that there is some person concealed underneath it who is waiting to assassinate him, his fancies may be dispelled or alleviated by allowing him to examine and convince himself that such is not actually the case. When he continues restless, he may very frequently be induced to keep quiet in bed, by holding out the prospect to him of a glass of beer after a time; patients suffering from this disease having a constant desire for porter or ale. He must be removed to a private room, where the greatest possible quiet must be observed; and in order that he may be under constant surveillance, a steady orderly ought to be in continual attendance to administer the medicine, to soothe his disturbed imagination, and prevent him from injuring himself or others.

When the patient has been guilty of acts of violence towards any of the attendants, the employment of restraint is frequently recommended; but I am of opinion that the efficacy of the strait-jacket in this disease is very questionable, and that it only tends to increase his dread that a plan has been formed against his life, or that it is but the commencement of a series of horrors to which he is to be subjected; thereby increasing the mental derangement which it never could have been expected to remove. In such cases, it will generally be found that the bowels are principally at fault; and that although it may sometimes be quite right to threaten the patient with the "jacket," we must hope to relieve their over-loaded state to be productive of more benefit than the employment of physical force. It is always best to act in a decided, although not harsh, manner; as the patient, notwithstanding his state of mental disorder, is always ready to take advantage of any leniency or pusillanimity which he may discover on the part of the Surgeon.

When we have once succeed in inducing sleep, a

favourable prognosis may generally be pronounced; but we must be careful not to disturb the patient for a very considerable time, nor be surprised if he should have an uninterrupted sleep of eighteen or twenty hours. In such a case, it will be advisable to arouse him; and then, his only complaints will generally be headache and weakness. Should he feel inclined to eat, he may be indulged in that respect; and under any circumstances he is to have his allowance of beer. After this the treatment becomes simple enough; all that is necessary to be done being in most cases merely to regulate the state of the bowels, and continue the patient's habitual stimulus, although of course in much smaller quantity than it was his custom to indulge in prior to the attack.

Notwithstanding our best directed endeavours, fatal cases of this as of all other diseases do sometimes occur; but by following the few simple instructions which I have just laid down, delirium tremens will, in most instances, be found to be by no means intractable.